CARNIVORE DIET COOKBOOK FOR SENIORS

80+ delicious and Simple Recipes to Fuel Your Body and Succeed in Your Golden Years

Alex kava

Copyright

No part of this publication may be reproduced, distributed, or transmitted in any form or by any means, including photocopying, recording, or other electronic or mechanical methods, without the prior written permission of the publisher, except in the case of brief quotations embodied in critical reviews and certain other noncommercial uses permitted by copyright law.

Table of contents

Introduction

In a small town nestled between rolling hills and lush forests, there lived a woman named Martha. She was not your typical senior citizen, for Martha possessed a secret that made her the envy of her peers. At 72 years old, she was the picture of health and vitality, and her secret was a cookbook with a peculiar title: **"Carnivore Diet Cookbook for Seniors."**

Martha's life had not always been this way. In her younger years, she had struggled with her health, battling various chronic illnesses, and obesity had been a constant companion. Her doctors had prescribed an array of medications, and her days were marked by pain, discomfort, and a sense of hopelessness. However, all of that changed one fateful day when she stumbled upon the intriguing book in a dusty corner of her local library.

The title had caught her eye, and she decided to borrow it, even though she had never considered herself a fan of diets. Little did she know that this book would transform her life in unimaginable ways.

Martha began to read the **"Carnivore Diet Cookbook for Seniors,"** authored by a nutritionist named Dr. Alex kava . The book advocated a diet that was primarily based on animal products – meat, fish, eggs, and dairy. It was a far cry from the conventional wisdom about balanced diets filled with fruits and vegetables. Intrigued by the bold claims and supported by a plethora of scientific studies cited in the book, Martha decided to give it a try.

With each page she turned, Martha learned about the remarkable health benefits of the carnivore diet. It promised increased energy, mental clarity, and relief from many of the ailments that had plagued her for years. It claimed to reduce inflammation, control blood sugar, and even aid in weight loss.

Armed with her newfound knowledge, Martha set out to transform her eating habits. She began by cleaning out her pantry of all the processed foods and sugary snacks. Instead, she filled her kitchen with the finest cuts of meat, fresh seafood, farm-fresh eggs, and high-quality dairy products. She also invested in a variety of herbs and spices to add flavor and variety to her carnivorous meals.

Martha's friends and family were initially skeptical of her radical diet change. They worried about her cholesterol levels and the supposed risks of consuming red meat. But Martha had faith in the science she had read, and she was determined to prove them wrong.

With dedication and creativity, she cooked up a storm in her kitchen. She marinated steaks in exotic spice blends, experimented with seafood recipes, and even concocted her own sauces to enhance the flavor of her meals. Over time, she noticed a remarkable change in her health. Her energy levels skyrocketed, and the chronic pain that had once plagued her gradually faded away.

Months turned into years, and Martha's carnivore diet became a way of life. She shed excess weight and found herself enjoying activities she had long abandoned, like hiking and dancing. Her blood pressure normalized, and her doctors reduced her medications. She felt decades younger and, as her friends began to notice her remarkable transformation, they too were intrigued by the **"Carnivore Diet Cookbook for Seniors."**

Inspired by Martha's success, a small group of seniors in her town formed a cooking club. They began to experiment with the carnivore diet, and each member brought their unique spin to the recipes they tried. They celebrated their newfound energy and vitality, sharing their stories and dishes at potluck dinners.

As the years passed, Martha's cookbook became a source of inspiration for many seniors, proving that age was not a barrier to experiencing a healthier and more vibrant life. It was a testament to the transformative power of knowledge and determination, illustrating that sometimes, a simple book title could open the door to a whole new chapter of life.

Chapter 1: Introduction to the Carnivore Diet

The Carnivore Diet, a dietary trend that has gained attention in recent years, has stirred controversy and curiosity alike. This unconventional eating regimen involves the exclusive consumption of animal products, primarily meat, and the complete exclusion of all plant-based foods. Advocates claim it offers a host of health benefits, from weight loss and improved mental clarity to reduced inflammation and better digestion. Critics, on the other hand, express concerns about the potential long-term health risks associated with a diet so devoid of plant nutrients.

In this introductory exploration, we delve into the origins, principles, and potential pros and cons of the Carnivore Diet, aiming to provide a comprehensive understanding of this increasingly popular but polarizing dietary approach.

A Historical Perspective

The Carnivore Diet isn't a recent invention; its roots can be traced back to various historical cultures and traditional diets. Indigenous Arctic communities, such as the Inuit and Eskimo, have subsisted on predominantly animal-based diets for centuries, relying on seals, whales, and fish for sustenance in environments where plant life is scarce. Similarly, the Maasai people in Africa are known for their consumption of animal products, particularly milk and meat.

Despite its historical context, the modern Carnivore Diet is significantly different from traditional practices. Contemporary followers of this diet often emphasize the consumption of high-quality, unprocessed animal products and exclude all plant-based foods, including fruits and vegetables.

The Principles of the Carnivore Diet

At its core, the Carnivore Diet is characterized by extreme simplicity - you eat only animal products.

The primary components of this diet typically include:

1. Meat: This forms the cornerstone of the Carnivore Diet. Followers predominantly consume red meat, but options can also include poultry, fish, and organ meats.

2. Fish and Seafood: Some individuals on the Carnivore Diet incorporate fish and seafood to diversify their animal-based protein sources.

3. Eggs: Eggs are a common part of the Carnivore Diet, providing a convenient source of protein and essential nutrients.

4. Dairy (optional): Some variations of the Carnivore Diet permit dairy products, such as butter and cheese. However, strict adherents exclude these.

5. Bone Broth: Bone broth, derived from simmering animal bones, is often included for its potential health benefits and nutrient content.

6. Animal Fat: Fat from animal sources, like tallow and lard, is encouraged as a primary source of energy.

The diet strictly excludes carbohydrates, fruits, vegetables, grains, legumes, and processed foods. Beverages are generally limited to water and certain animal-based options, such as bone broth and beef tallow tea.

The Controversy Surrounding the Carnivore Diet

The Carnivore Diet's polarizing nature stems from the extreme restrictions it imposes on food choices and its deviation from conventional nutritional wisdom. Proponents of the diet argue that it offers a range of potential benefits, including weight loss, improved mental focus, and reduced inflammation. Some even claim it can alleviate chronic health conditions like autoimmune diseases.

Critics, however, express serious reservations about the diet's long-term safety and nutritional completeness. They highlight concerns about nutrient deficiencies, such as fiber, vitamins, and minerals, which are typically found in plant-based foods. The lack of dietary diversity on the Carnivore Diet has raised questions about potential health risks over time.

In the subsequent sections, we will delve into the potential benefits and drawbacks of the Carnivore Diet, as well as the existing scientific evidence surrounding this dietary approach. Whether you're considering adopting this diet, are merely curious about its effects, or seeking a balanced viewpoint, this exploration will provide valuable insights into the controversial world of the Carnivore Diet.

Understanding the Carnivore Diet

In recent years, dietary trends and fads have proliferated, offering a wide array of options for those seeking to improve their health, lose weight, or optimize their nutrition. Among these various diets, the Carnivore Diet has gained popularity as a unique and controversial approach to eating. Unlike many mainstream diets that emphasize a balanced intake of fruits, vegetables, and grains, the Carnivore Diet is a nutritional regimen that revolves around one primary food group: animal products. This minimalist approach to eating has sparked curiosity, debate, and polarized opinions among health enthusiasts and experts. In this exploration of the Carnivore Diet, we will delve into the principles, historical context, scientific evidence, and potential benefits and risks associated with this unconventional dietary choice.

The Carnivore Diet, sometimes referred to as the All-Meat Diet, is a dietary regimen that promotes the exclusive consumption of animal products. These animal products typically include meat, fish, and animal-derived fats, such as butter and tallow, while excluding all plant-based foods, such as fruits, vegetables, grains, legumes, and even processed foods. This extreme departure from conventional dietary guidelines is based on the premise that humans evolved as carnivorous creatures and, as such, are best adapted to thrive on an all-meat diet.

The origins of the Carnivore Diet can be traced back to the controversial work of Dr. Vilhjalmur Stefansson, an Arctic explorer and anthropologist, in the early 20th century. Stefansson lived with the Inuit people in Canada's Arctic and observed their exceptional health and vitality despite subsisting primarily on animal-based diets. His experiences and studies laid the foundation for the argument that an all-meat diet could offer numerous health benefits. However, it's worth noting that Stefansson's findings were met with skepticism and were considered by many to be anecdotal and incomplete.

Over the years, the Carnivore Diet has evolved and garnered a dedicated following, particularly within the online health and fitness communities. Advocates claim that adopting this diet can lead to a wide range of health benefits, including weight loss, improved mental clarity, increased energy, and relief from various health conditions, such as autoimmune diseases and digestive disorders. These claims have sparked considerable interest among those who are disillusioned with traditional dietary recommendations and are seeking alternative approaches to achieve optimal health.

As with any dietary trend, the Carnivore Diet is not without controversy and skepticism. Many health professionals and nutritional experts express concerns about the diet's lack of diversity and the potential for nutrient deficiencies, particularly in vitamins, minerals, and fiber. Critics argue that relying solely on animal products may lead to imbalances in the diet and long-term health risks, such as heart disease, kidney problems, and gastrointestinal issues.

Understanding the Carnivore Diet requires a balanced examination of both its proponents' claims and the scientific evidence surrounding it. This exploration will delve deeper into the principles and potential benefits of the Carnivore Diet, as well as the concerns and risks associated with this highly restrictive eating pattern. By providing a comprehensive view of this unconventional dietary choice, readers can make informed decisions about whether or not the Carnivore Diet aligns with their personal health and wellness goals.

Benefits of the Carnivore Diet for Seniors

The Carnivore Diet, a nutritional approach that centers on the exclusive consumption of animal products, has garnered widespread attention for its potential health benefits. While it remains a topic of debate and scrutiny, one demographic that has shown particular interest in the Carnivore Diet is seniors. As individuals age, their nutritional needs often change, and they may be seeking dietary options that promote better health, vitality, and quality of life. In this exploration of the Carnivore Diet, we will focus on its potential benefits for seniors, offering insight into how this unconventional eating pattern may address specific age-related concerns and promote overall well-being.

Aging is an inevitable part of life, accompanied by a range of physiological changes and health challenges. Seniors may experience a decline in muscle mass, bone density, and metabolic rate, as well as an increased risk of chronic conditions like cardiovascular disease, diabetes, and osteoporosis. As such, the role of nutrition in the lives of older individuals becomes increasingly important. The Carnivore Diet presents itself as a unique option that seniors are considering to address some of these age-related issues.

One of the primary claims made by proponents of the Carnivore Diet is that it can support muscle preservation and potentially even promote muscle growth. This is particularly appealing to seniors, as the gradual loss of muscle mass, known as sarcopenia, is a common concern with aging. The diet's emphasis on protein-rich animal foods, such as lean cuts of meat, fish, and eggs, provides essential amino acids necessary for maintaining and building muscle. This may be especially advantageous for seniors who wish to sustain their strength and independence as they age.

The Carnivore Diet also tends to be low in carbohydrates and does not include high-glycemic foods, which can lead to blood sugar spikes. For seniors at risk of or managing type 2 diabetes or metabolic syndrome, this low-carb aspect of the diet may help stabilize blood sugar levels and reduce the need for medication. Furthermore, it could contribute to weight management, as excess weight is a risk factor for various age-related conditions, including heart disease and joint problems.

Another potential benefit for seniors is the diet's simplicity and ease of digestion. With age, the digestive system may become more sensitive, and some individuals may experience discomfort or allergies related to certain foods. The Carnivore Diet eliminates many common allergens, such as gluten and lactose, and consists of easily digestible animal products. This could help seniors avoid digestive issues and enjoy their meals without worry.

However, it's essential to acknowledge that the Carnivore Diet is not without its share of controversy and concerns, especially for older adults. Critics argue that the exclusion of fruits and vegetables, which are rich in vitamins, minerals, and fiber, could lead to nutrient deficiencies and digestive problems in the long run. Furthermore, the potential risks associated with a diet high in saturated fats, like those found in red meat and dairy products, must be carefully considered.

In this exploration of the Carnivore Diet, we will provide a balanced view of the potential benefits and risks for seniors who may be considering this dietary approach. It's crucial to remember that individual health and nutritional needs can vary, and what works for one person may not be suitable for another. As with any diet, it's advisable for seniors to consult with a healthcare professional before making significant changes to their eating habits. By examining the potential advantages and drawbacks of the Carnivore Diet for seniors, we aim to empower individuals to make informed choices about their health and well-being as they age.

Safety Considerations and Precautions

The Carnivore Diet, a dietary regimen that primarily consists of animal products while excluding plant-based foods, has gained attention for its potential health benefits. However, this highly restrictive approach to nutrition is not without controversy and safety concerns. Before embarking on the Carnivore Diet, it is essential to consider the potential risks and precautions associated with this unconventional eating pattern. In this exploration, we will delve into safety considerations and offer guidance to help individuals make informed decisions about whether the Carnivore Diet is right for them.

While the Carnivore Diet has attracted a dedicated following of proponents who extol its potential health benefits, it has also faced criticism and skepticism from health professionals, nutrition experts, and scientific communities. One of the primary concerns surrounding this diet is the lack of dietary diversity. Excluding fruits, vegetables, grains, and legumes means that followers of the Carnivore Diet may miss out on essential vitamins, minerals, and fiber that are abundant in plant-based foods. This restriction raises concerns about nutrient deficiencies and the long-term health consequences of excluding these vital nutrients from one's diet.

Furthermore, the diet's emphasis on animal products, particularly red meat, can lead to an increased intake of saturated fats and cholesterol. Consuming excessive amounts of saturated fats has long been associated with an increased risk of heart disease and other cardiovascular issues. Individuals with a history of heart problems or those at risk for heart disease should exercise extreme caution when considering the Carnivore Diet.

Digestive health is another significant consideration. The sudden switch to an all-meat diet may result in digestive discomfort for some individuals. Fiber, which is found in plant foods, plays a crucial role in regulating bowel movements and maintaining gut health. A diet devoid of fiber could lead to constipation and other digestive issues. Additionally, some people may experience adverse reactions to certain types of meat or animal products, such as dairy, which can lead to food allergies or sensitivities.

Ketosis, a metabolic state where the body primarily burns fat for energy, is often a goal of the Carnivore Diet. While ketosis can be a safe and effective way to burn excess body fat, it can also result in side effects known as the "keto flu." Symptoms may include headaches, fatigue, nausea, and dizziness. Seniors, individuals with certain medical conditions, and those with specific dietary requirements should be particularly cautious about entering a state of ketosis without medical supervision.

Individual variations in health, metabolism, and dietary preferences should not be overlooked when considering the Carnivore Diet. Before making any significant dietary changes, it is essential to consult with a healthcare professional or registered dietitian. They can provide personalized guidance and ensure that the diet aligns with your unique nutritional needs and goals. Additionally, regular health check-ups and monitoring are crucial when following any specialized diet, such as the Carnivore Diet, to detect any potential health issues early on.

While the Carnivore Diet has sparked interest and debate in the world of nutrition, it is vital to consider the safety considerations and precautions associated with this highly restrictive eating pattern. Potential risks such as nutrient deficiencies, digestive problems, and cardiovascular concerns must be carefully weighed against the perceived benefits of the diet. Before embarking on the Carnivore Diet, it is advisable to seek guidance from healthcare professionals who can help individuals make informed decisions about their dietary choices and ensure that they prioritize their health and well-being.

Chapter 2: Getting Started

The Carnivore Diet is a dietary approach that has gained popularity in recent years, promoting the consumption of animal-based foods while excluding plant-based foods entirely. This extreme diet has its proponents and critics, and before you consider embarking on this journey, it's crucial to understand the basics and potential risks involved. In this guide, we will explore the fundamental principles of the Carnivore Diet and provide insights on how to get started safely and effectively.

What is the Carnivore Diet?

The Carnivore Diet is a diet that emphasizes the exclusive consumption of animal-based foods, primarily meat, and animal-derived products. Advocates of the diet claim that it can offer various health benefits, including weight loss, improved mental clarity, and relief from certain health conditions.

Key Principles of the Carnivore Diet:

1. Animal-Based Foods: The foundation of the Carnivore Diet is meat. Beef, lamb, pork, and poultry are commonly included, but some individuals also incorporate other animal products like fish and dairy, depending on their personal preferences and tolerance.

2. No Plant-Based Foods: Unlike many other diets, the Carnivore Diet excludes all plant-based foods, including vegetables, fruits, grains, legumes, and nuts. This strict restriction is one of the most distinguishing features of the diet.

3. Limited to No Carbohydrates: Carbohydrate intake is minimized to virtually zero on the Carnivore Diet. This means no bread, pasta, rice, or any other sources of carbohydrates are allowed.

4. Focus on Fatty Cuts of Meat: The diet encourages the consumption of fatty cuts of meat to provide essential nutrients and energy. This often means eating ribeye steaks, bacon, and other high-fat meats.

5. Water and Salt: Staying hydrated and maintaining adequate salt intake are essential for Carnivore Diet practitioners. This helps prevent electrolyte imbalances and other potential health issues.

Getting Started with the Carnivore Diet:

1. Consult a Healthcare Professional: Before starting any new diet, especially one as restrictive as the Carnivore Diet, it's essential to consult a healthcare professional or registered dietitian. They can assess your health and dietary needs to ensure that this approach is suitable for you.

2. Research and Educate Yourself: Familiarize yourself with the principles and guidelines of the Carnivore Diet. Read books, articles, and testimonials from individuals who have followed this diet to understand what to expect.

3. Plan Your Meals: Create a meal plan that includes a variety of animal-based foods, such as beef, pork, poultry, and fish. Consider your preferences and dietary requirements while planning your meals.

4. Monitor Your Health: Throughout your journey on the Carnivore Diet, it's essential to keep an eye on your health. Pay attention to your energy levels, digestion, and any potential side effects, and consult with a healthcare professional if you experience any concerning symptoms.

5. Gradual Transition: If you are currently following a standard diet, consider gradually transitioning into the Carnivore Diet. Slowly reduce your intake of plant-based foods while increasing your consumption of animal products.

6. Be Mindful of Nutrient Intake: Ensure you are obtaining all essential nutrients from your diet. Vitamins and minerals such as vitamin C, fiber, and antioxidants are typically absent from the Carnivore

Diet, so you may need to consider supplements or specialized foods to address potential deficiencies.

7. Listen to Your Body: The Carnivore Diet may not be suitable for everyone. Pay attention to how your body responds to the diet, and be prepared to adjust or modify it based on your individual needs and preferences.

The Carnivore Diet is a highly restrictive dietary approach that advocates claim can have various health benefits. However, it is essential to approach this diet with caution and thorough research. Always consult a healthcare professional before making significant dietary changes, and be mindful of your body's response to the diet. Ultimately, the Carnivore Diet is not for everyone, and its long-term effects and safety are still subjects of ongoing debate and research.

Setting Up Your Carnivore Kitchen

Embarking on the Carnivore Diet means making a significant dietary shift towards an animal-based eating pattern. To succeed in this journey, it's essential to set up your Carnivore kitchen thoughtfully. In this guide, we'll explore the key steps to create a Carnivore-friendly kitchen, which will make meal preparation easier and more convenient as you follow this unique diet.

1. Clear Your Kitchen of Plant-Based Foods

Before you start building a Carnivore kitchen, it's crucial to eliminate plant-based foods that are not compliant with the diet. This includes grains, vegetables, fruits, nuts, and legumes. Go through your pantry, refrigerator, and freezer, and remove any non-Carnivore items.

2. Stock Up on Animal-Based Foods

Since animal-based foods are the core of the Carnivore Diet, you'll need to have a variety of meat and animal-derived products on hand. Here are some essential items to stock up on:

  - **Beef:** Ground beef, steaks, roasts, and organ meats like liver.
  - **Pork:** Pork chops, bacon, and other cuts.
  - **Poultry:** Chicken thighs, wings, and other parts.
  - **Lamb:** Lamb chops, ground lamb, and organ meats.
  - **Fish:** Salmon, mackerel, and other fatty fish.
  - **Eggs:** A great source of nutrients and protein.
  - **Dairy (optional):** If you choose to include dairy, opt for full-fat options like butter, heavy cream, and cheese.

3. Invest in Quality Cooking Equipment

To make cooking on the Carnivore Diet more efficient and enjoyable, invest in quality cooking equipment. Here are some items that can be especially helpful:

- **Cast Iron Skillet:** Perfect for searing steaks and other meats.

- **Meat Thermometer:** Ensure your meat is cooked to your preferred level of doneness.

- **Grill or Smoker (optional):** If you enjoy outdoor cooking, a grill or smoker can add variety to your meals.

- **Oven-Safe Baking Dish:** Useful for roasting meats or preparing casseroles.

- **Food Scale:** Helpful for portion control and tracking your protein intake.

- **Sharp Knives:** Invest in high-quality knives for slicing and cutting meat.

4. Plan for Food Storage

Proper food storage is essential to maintain the freshness and safety of your Carnivore foods. Consider the following storage options:

- **Refrigerator and Freezer:** Ensure you have enough space to store your meat and animal products. Invest in quality freezer-safe bags or containers for portioning and storing your meat.

- **Airtight Containers:** Use airtight containers to keep your meat fresh in the refrigerator.

- **Vacuum Sealer (optional):** A vacuum sealer can help extend the shelf life of your meat by removing air from the packaging.

5. Learn About Cooking Techniques

While the Carnivore Diet may seem straightforward in terms of food choices, mastering cooking techniques is essential for creating enjoyable meals. Learn how to grill, pan-sear, roast, and slow-cook different cuts of meat to add variety and flavor to your diet.

6. Seasonings and Spices

Though the Carnivore Diet primarily focuses on animal-based foods, you can enhance the flavor of your dishes with various spices and seasonings. Common Carnivore-friendly options include salt, pepper, and herbs like rosemary and thyme. Be sure to check the ingredient lists on spice blends to avoid hidden additives or non-compliant ingredients.

Setting up your Carnivore kitchen is a crucial step in successfully adopting the Carnivore Diet. By clearing your kitchen of non-compliant foods, stocking up on quality animal-based products, and acquiring the necessary cooking equipment, you'll be well-prepared to enjoy the benefits of this unique dietary approach. With careful planning and knowledge of Carnivore cooking techniques, you can make your kitchen a haven for delicious and nutritious meat-centric meals.

Grocery Shopping Tips for Seniors

Grocery shopping is a routine task for most people, but for seniors, it can present unique challenges. As we age, it becomes increasingly important to make informed and convenient choices when it comes to shopping for groceries. This guide provides practical tips to help seniors navigate the grocery store with ease, maintain a balanced diet, and enhance their overall well-being.

1. Plan Ahead

Before heading to the grocery store, take some time to plan your shopping trip:

  - **Create a shopping list:** Jot down the items you need, focusing on essential and nutritious foods like fruits, vegetables, lean proteins, and whole grains.
  - **Check your pantry:** Review your existing inventory to avoid unnecessary purchases and ensure you're replenishing what you need.
  - **Schedule your trip:** Choose a time that suits you best, when the store is less crowded, to minimize stress and waiting in line.

2. Shop Online

Many grocery stores now offer online shopping and home delivery services, making it incredibly convenient for seniors. This option saves you the physical effort of navigating the store and carrying heavy bags. Consider exploring this alternative if it's available in your area.

3. Opt for Smaller Stores

Larger supermarkets can be overwhelming and physically demanding. Smaller, neighborhood grocery stores often have shorter aisles and fewer crowds, making them more senior-friendly. Plus, they may offer a more personalized and relaxed shopping experience.

4. Use a Shopping Cart or Basket

Using a shopping cart or basket provides support and stability while you move around the store. It can also help distribute the weight of your groceries, reducing the strain on your body.

5. Choose Nutrient-Rich Foods

When shopping, prioritize nutrient-rich foods that promote health and well-being. Some essential items include:

- **Fresh fruits and vegetables:** These provide vitamins, fiber, and antioxidants.

- **Lean proteins:** Select lean cuts of meat, poultry, fish, or plant-based proteins like beans and tofu.

- **Whole grains:** Look for whole-grain bread, pasta, and cereals to support heart and digestive health.

- **Dairy or dairy alternatives:** Include low-fat milk, yogurt, or lactose-free options for calcium and vitamin D.

6. Read Labels

Pay close attention to food labels, especially for products with a long shelf life. Look for low-sodium, low-sugar, and low-fat options. Opt for items with fewer additives and preservatives, as these can impact health, particularly in seniors.

7. Embrace Convenience

While fresh, whole foods are ideal, convenience items can save time and effort. Consider items like pre-cut vegetables, frozen fruits, and pre-cooked proteins. Just be cautious of added sugars, sodium, or unhealthy fats in some convenience foods.

8. Mind Your Budget

Seniors on fixed incomes should be mindful of their budget. Look for sales, discounts, and coupons to maximize savings. Buying store-brand items can also be a cost-effective choice.

9. Stay Hydrated

Don't forget to include beverages on your shopping list. Water is crucial for hydration, and herbal teas or low-sugar, low-sodium juices can be tasty and hydrating alternatives.

10. Ask for Assistance

If you need help, don't hesitate to ask a store employee for assistance with reaching items on high shelves, or ask for help with carrying groceries to your car.

Grocery shopping is a necessary part of life, and with these tips, seniors can make the experience more manageable and enjoyable. Prioritizing a balanced diet, planning your trips, and considering convenient options will help ensure you maintain a healthy and nutritious diet, which is vital for your well-being as you age.

Meal Planning and Preparation Techniques

Meal planning and preparation are essential skills for anyone looking to eat healthily, save time, and reduce stress in the kitchen. This guide aims to help you get started with meal planning and provide practical techniques to streamline your cooking process, whether you're a novice or an experienced cook.

Benefits of Meal Planning and Preparation

Before diving into the techniques, let's highlight some of the benefits of meal planning and preparation:

1. Healthier Eating: When you plan your meals in advance, you're more likely to make nutritious choices and avoid the temptation of fast food or unhealthy snacks.

2. Time-Saving: By dedicating time to plan and prepare your meals, you can save valuable time during busy weekdays.

3. Cost-Effective: Meal planning can help you reduce food waste and make the most of your groceries, ultimately saving you money.

4. Reduced Stress: Knowing what you're going to eat and having ingredients ready in advance can alleviate stress and indecision when it's time to cook.

Now, let's explore the techniques to get started with meal planning and preparation:

1. Set Realistic Goals

Begin with clear and attainable objectives. Consider how many meals you want to plan for each week, taking into account your schedule and dietary preferences. Start with planning for just a few meals and gradually expand as you become more comfortable with the process.

2. Choose Your Planning Tools

Select a method that suits your style. You can use a physical planner, a dedicated app, or a simple digital calendar to organize your meal plans. There are various meal planning apps available that can help you create shopping lists and store your recipes.

3. Create a Weekly Menu

Plan your meals for the week ahead. Include breakfast, lunch, dinner, and snacks. Be sure to incorporate a variety of foods to ensure a balanced diet, and consider your dietary restrictions or preferences.

4. Make a Shopping List

Once your weekly menu is complete, create a shopping list that includes all the ingredients you'll need for your planned meals. This will help you avoid impulsive purchases and ensure you have everything on hand.

5. Batch Cooking

Consider batch cooking, where you prepare multiple servings of a meal at once. This can save you time and effort, and you can freeze extra portions for future meals. For instance, you can batch cook a big pot of soup, chili, or stew.

6. Prep Ingredients in Advance

Before you start cooking, take time to prepare and chop ingredients. This can be done on the weekend or a less busy day. Having prepped vegetables, grains, and proteins on hand makes weeknight cooking much easier and quicker.

7. Use a Slow Cooker or Instant Pot

These kitchen appliances can be invaluable for meal planning. You can set up your meal in the morning and come home to a hot, ready-to-eat dinner. They're perfect for stews, soups, and even some one-pot pasta dishes.

8. Embrace Freezer-Friendly Meals

Prepare dishes that freeze well, such as lasagna, casseroles, or marinated meats. These can be stored in portioned containers and thawed when needed.

9. Leftovers Are Your Friend

Don't underestimate the power of leftovers. Make extra portions during dinner, and you'll have a convenient lunch for the next day. You can also repurpose leftovers into new dishes, like turning roasted vegetables into a frittata or chicken into a sandwich.

10. Be Flexible

Remember that meal planning is a tool to make your life easier, not a strict regimen. Be flexible and open to adjusting your plan if needed. Life can be unpredictable, and sometimes plans change.

Meal planning and preparation techniques can significantly enhance your eating habits, save you time, and reduce stress in the kitchen. By setting realistic goals, choosing the right tools, and embracing batch cooking and other time-saving strategies, you'll be well on your way to a more organized and efficient approach to meal planning and preparation. Enjoy the benefits of healthier, homemade meals with less effort and stress.

Chapter 3: Breakfast and Brunch Delights

Breakfast and brunch are not just meals; they're delightful experiences that set the tone for the rest of your day. Whether you prefer a quick and simple breakfast on a busy morning or a leisurely brunch on a lazy weekend, there's a wide array of delectable dishes to choose from. These morning delights are more than just sustenance; they're a celebration of flavors, textures, and cultural diversity.

1. Classic Breakfast Favorites:

  - **Pancakes:** Fluffy and golden, pancakes are a beloved morning treat. Stack them high and drizzle with maple syrup, or customize them with toppings like berries, chocolate chips, or nuts.

  - **Waffles:** Crisp on the outside, tender on the inside, waffles offer a perfect canvas for your creativity. Top them with fresh fruit, whipped cream, or a dollop of Nutella for an indulgent twist.

- **French Toast:** Thick slices of bread soaked in a sweet custard, fried to perfection, and dusted with powdered sugar. It's a timeless classic that combines a hint of sweetness with a satisfying, custardy texture.

2. Savory Delights:

- **Eggs Benedict:** A true brunch classic, eggs Benedict features poached eggs, Canadian bacon, and hollandaise sauce atop a toasted English muffin. It's a harmonious blend of flavors and textures.

- **Omelettes:** Whisked eggs filled with an assortment of ingredients like cheese, vegetables, and meats, omelettes offer endless possibilities for customization.

- **Avocado Toast:** A trendy and healthy option, avocado toast combines creamy slices of avocado on toasted bread, often garnished with various toppings like tomatoes, poached eggs, or feta cheese.

3. International Flavors:

- **Chilaquiles:** A Mexican breakfast delight, chilaquiles consist of crispy tortilla chips smothered in red or green salsa, then topped with cheese, sour cream, and sometimes fried eggs.

- **Dim Sum:** A Chinese brunch tradition, dim sum offers a variety of steamed or fried dumplings, buns, and small plates like pork buns, spring rolls, and shrimp dumplings.

- **Croissants:** This quintessential French pastry, when filled with ham and cheese, transforms into a delightful breakfast sandwich. Pair it with a latte, and you've got a classic French breakfast.

4. Healthier Options:

- **Greek Yogurt Parfait:** Layered with granola, fresh berries, and honey, Greek yogurt parfaits are a nutritious and satisfying way to start your day.

- **Smoothie Bowls:** Blended with fruits, vegetables, and your choice of toppings, smoothie bowls are a colorful and refreshing breakfast or brunch option.

- **Acai Bowls:** Hailing from Brazil, acai bowls feature acai berry puree topped with granola, fresh fruit, and a drizzle of honey, providing a burst of antioxidants.

5. Specialty Coffees and Teas:

- **Espresso:** For those who need a quick caffeine boost, a shot of espresso is the go-to choice. It can be enjoyed on its own or used as a base for various coffee beverages.

- **Chai Latte:** A spiced tea latte, combining black tea with aromatic spices and steamed milk, is a cozy and fragrant option.

- **Matcha Latte:** Made from finely ground green tea leaves, matcha lattes offer a vibrant green color and a unique earthy flavor.

Breakfast and brunch are not only about satisfying your hunger but also an opportunity to relish diverse and delightful flavors. Whether you prefer sweet or savory, traditional or exotic, there's a breakfast or brunch delight to suit every palate. So, explore, savor, and make the most of these morning culinary delights to kickstart your day with a smile.

Scrumptious Steak and Eggs

Steak and eggs is a classic breakfast and brunch dish that combines the rich, hearty flavors of a perfectly cooked steak with the creamy texture and protein punch of eggs. This dish has been a beloved indulgence for many, appealing to those who appreciate a savory start to their day. Let's explore the delightful combination of scrumptious steak and eggs.

The Perfect Steak:

A key element of this dish is the steak, which can vary in cuts and preparations, depending on personal preference. Here are some popular options:

1. Ribeye: Known for its marbling, ribeye steaks are tender, juicy, and rich in flavor. They are often pan-seared to perfection, creating a caramelized crust.

2. New York Strip: This cut offers a balance of tenderness and a beefy flavor. It's often seasoned with salt, pepper, and maybe a touch of garlic before grilling or searing.

3. Filet Mignon: Renowned for its tenderness, filet mignon is usually cooked to a medium-rare or rare state, allowing its natural flavors to shine through.

4. Sirloin: A more budget-friendly option, sirloin steaks are leaner but still flavorful when seasoned and cooked to the desired doneness.

Eggs in Various Styles:
The choice of eggs to accompany the steak can add a different dimension to the dish:

1. Sunny-Side-Up: A classic choice, sunny-side-up eggs are fried with the yolks intact, creating a runny, golden center that complements the steak's richness.

2. Scrambled: Scrambled eggs, cooked with a touch of butter or cream, provide a fluffy, creamy contrast to the steak's texture.

3. Poached: Poached eggs, with their silky, runny yolks, can be an elegant addition to this hearty dish.

Accompaniments:

To enhance the overall experience, consider adding some flavorful side dishes and garnishes:

1. Hash Browns: Crispy, golden-brown hash browns are a classic pairing that provides a satisfying crunch.

2. Sautéed Mushrooms: The earthy flavors of sautéed mushrooms can complement the richness of the steak and add depth to the dish.

3. Sauce: A drizzle of Béarnaise sauce, mushroom gravy, or a simple steak sauce can elevate the flavors even further.

Serving Options:

Steak and eggs can be served in various ways:

1. On a Plate: A classic presentation with the steak and eggs placed side by side, often garnished with herbs and seasonings.

2. Breakfast Burrito: Roll the steak and eggs inside a tortilla for a portable and satisfying breakfast option.

3. Open-Faced Sandwich: Place the steak and eggs on a slice of toasted bread or an English muffin for a hearty sandwich.

4. Benedict-style: A twist on the classic Eggs Benedict, substitute the Canadian bacon with a steak and top with hollandaise sauce.

Steak and eggs are a decadent breakfast or brunch choice that combines the robust flavors of a well-cooked steak with the lusciousness of eggs in various styles. The versatility of this dish allows for personalization, making it a delightful and indulgent option to start your day with a burst of flavor and energy. Whether you prefer your steak rare, medium, or well-done, there's no denying the scrumptious delight that this pairing brings to the table.

Bacon-Wrapped Avocado Boats

Bacon-wrapped avocado boats are a mouthwatering breakfast and brunch delight that brings together the rich, creamy goodness of avocados with the savory, smoky flavor of crispy bacon. This dish is a perfect combination of textures and flavors that is not only satisfying but also a treat for the senses. Let's dive into the wonderful world of bacon-wrapped avocado boats.

Ingredients for Bacon-Wrapped Avocado Boats:

1. Avocados: Choose ripe, firm avocados, which will serve as the base of this dish. Their creamy texture pairs wonderfully with crispy bacon.

2. Bacon: Opt for high-quality bacon slices to ensure that they crisp up nicely during cooking. You can use regular or thick-cut bacon, depending on your preference.

3. Eggs (optional): If you want to add some protein to this dish, consider scooping out a bit of avocado to create space for an egg. A poached or fried egg nestled in the avocado boat can be a delightful addition.

4. Seasonings: You can use a variety of seasonings, such as salt, pepper, garlic powder, or even a pinch of paprika, to add flavor to the avocados.

Preparation:

1. Halve and Pit the Avocados: Carefully cut the avocados in half lengthwise, remove the pits, and scoop out a small portion of the flesh to create a hollowed-out space for your toppings. Season the avocado halves with your choice of seasonings.

2. Wrap with Bacon: Wrap each avocado half with bacon slices, ensuring that the bacon covers the entire outer surface. You can secure the bacon with toothpicks if needed.

3. Egg Option: If you'd like to add eggs, create a small well in the scooped-out avocado, and gently crack an egg into it. Season the egg with salt and pepper.

Cooking Methods:

1. Oven-Baking: Place the bacon-wrapped avocado halves on a baking sheet and bake them in a preheated oven at 350°F (175°C) for about 15-20 minutes, or until the bacon is crispy and the avocados are tender.

2. Grilling: You can also cook bacon-wrapped avocado boats on a grill. Just make sure to use indirect heat to prevent excessive charring.

3. Skillet: Cook them in a skillet over medium heat, turning them frequently to ensure that the bacon cooks evenly.

Serving and Garnishes:

Once your bacon-wrapped avocado boats are cooked to perfection, it's time to serve them. Here are some garnishes and serving suggestions to consider:

1. Fresh Herbs: Sprinkle your creation with fresh herbs like chopped cilantro, parsley, or chives to add a burst of color and freshness.

2. Salsa: A drizzle of salsa, whether it's a classic tomato salsa or a fruity mango salsa, can add a zesty kick to the dish.

3. Lime Wedges: Serve with lime wedges on the side to provide a citrusy contrast to the richness of the avocados and bacon.

4. Hot Sauce: For those who enjoy a little heat, hot sauce or chili flakes can be the perfect condiment.

bacon-wrapped avocado boats are a delightful breakfast and brunch option that combines the lusciousness of avocados with the smoky, salty goodness of bacon. Whether you choose to include eggs or experiment with different seasonings and toppings, this dish is a crowd-pleaser that's perfect for those looking to start their day with a burst of flavor and indulgence. Try it for your next brunch gathering, and you'll surely leave your guests craving for more.

Sausage and Cheese Omelette

A sausage and cheese omelette is a quintessential breakfast and brunch delight that marries the hearty, savory flavors of sausage and the melty goodness of cheese in a fluffy, folded egg package. Omelettes are incredibly versatile, allowing you to personalize them with various ingredients to suit your taste. Here, we'll explore the classic combination of sausage and cheese in this satisfying breakfast dish.

Ingredients for a Sausage and Cheese Omelette:

1. Eggs: The base of any omelette is, of course, eggs. You'll typically need two to three large eggs per omelette, depending on your appetite.

2. Sausage: You can use your favorite type of sausage, whether it's pork, chicken, turkey, or a plant-based sausage for a vegetarian version. Cook the sausage and crumble or slice it before adding it to the omelette.

3. Cheese: Choose a cheese that melts well for the ultimate oozing, cheesy goodness. Cheddar, Swiss, Monterey Jack, or mozzarella are popular choices.

4. Seasonings: A pinch of salt, pepper, and other preferred seasonings like garlic powder or fresh herbs can enhance the flavors.

5. Butter or Oil: Use a small amount of butter or oil to coat the skillet and prevent sticking.

Steps to Make a Sausage and Cheese Omelette:

1. Whisk the Eggs: Crack the eggs into a bowl, add a pinch of salt and pepper, and beat them until well combined. You can also add a dash of milk or cream for extra fluffiness.

2. Cook the Sausage: In a separate skillet, cook the sausage until it's browned and fully cooked. Remove the sausage from the skillet and set it aside.

3. Heat the Skillet: Place a non-stick skillet over medium-low heat and add a small amount of butter or oil. Swirl it around to coat the bottom of the skillet.

4. Pour and Cook the Eggs: Once the butter is melted and hot, pour the beaten eggs into the skillet. Allow them to cook undisturbed for a minute or two until the edges start to set.

5. Add Sausage and Cheese: Sprinkle the cooked sausage and shredded cheese over one half of the omelette.

6. Fold and Serve: Carefully fold the other half of the omelette over the sausage and cheese, creating a semi-circle shape. Cook for an additional minute or until the cheese melts.

7. Slide and Plate: Gently slide the omelette onto a plate, and it's ready to serve.

Variations and Garnishes:

You can customize your sausage and cheese omelette with various ingredients to suit your preferences. Here are some ideas:

- **Vegetables:** Add sautéed onions, bell peppers, mushrooms, or spinach for extra flavor and nutrition.
- **Herbs:** Fresh herbs like chives, parsley, or cilantro can provide a burst of freshness.
- **Hot Sauce:** Drizzle with hot sauce for a spicy kick.
- **Sour Cream or Salsa:** Serve with a dollop of sour cream or a side of salsa for added zest.

Sausage and cheese omelettes are a delightful way to start your day with a hearty and satisfying meal. The combination of savory sausage and gooey cheese enveloped in fluffy, perfectly cooked eggs is a breakfast and brunch classic that never goes out of style. Whether you enjoy it on its own or with a side of toast or hash browns, this dish is sure to leave you with a smile on your face.

Chapter 4: Lunch and Dinner Favorites

Lunch and dinner are two of the most anticipated meals of the day, and they offer a wonderful opportunity to savor delicious and satisfying dishes. Whether you're a food enthusiast or simply someone who enjoys a good meal, there's no shortage of lunch and dinner favorites to explore. From traditional comfort foods to gourmet creations, the world of culinary delights is vast and diverse.

Let's delve into some popular lunch and dinner favorites that people around the world enjoy:

1. Sandwiches:

Sandwiches are a classic and versatile choice for lunch. From a simple yet satisfying peanut butter and jelly sandwich to gourmet creations like a lobster roll or a Reuben, there's a sandwich for every taste. Whether you prefer your sandwich warm or cold, they make for a quick and convenient meal.

2. Pizza:

Pizza is a universal favorite. The combination of a crispy crust, rich tomato sauce, melted cheese, and a variety of toppings makes it an irresistible choice for dinner. From classic Margherita to loaded supreme pizzas, the options are endless, and it's a go-to comfort food for many.

3. Burgers:

Burgers are a symbol of American fast food, but they've become a global sensation. A juicy beef patty or a plant-based alternative, sandwiched between soft buns and dressed with a variety of condiments, is a beloved choice for lunch or dinner. You can customize your burger with toppings like lettuce, tomatoes, onions, cheese, and more.

4. Sushi:

Sushi is a Japanese delicacy that has gained immense popularity worldwide. Sushi rolls, sashimi, and nigiri offer a wide range of flavors and textures.

Fresh seafood, rice, and seaweed are combined with precision, and soy sauce, wasabi, and pickled ginger add depth to the experience.

5. Pasta:

Pasta is a comfort food that has deep roots in Italian cuisine but is enjoyed globally. From spaghetti with marinara sauce to creamy fettuccine Alfredo and rich lasagna, pasta dishes come in various forms, and the combinations of sauces and toppings are endless.

6. Tacos:

Tacos are a Mexican staple that has found its way into the hearts of people worldwide. Soft or crispy tortillas filled with an array of ingredients such as seasoned meat, beans, cheese, salsa, and fresh vegetables create a symphony of flavors in each bite.

7. Curry:

Curry dishes, originating from India but embraced by many cultures, are a hearty and aromatic choice for dinner. Whether it's a spicy Thai green curry, a creamy Indian butter chicken, or a Japanese katsu curry, the diverse world of curries offers something for everyone.

8. Grilled Steak:

For those who love a hearty and meaty dinner, a perfectly grilled steak is a top choice. The smoky, charred flavor of a well-cooked steak, whether it's a ribeye, sirloin, or filet mignon, is a culinary delight. Pair it with sides like mashed potatoes or grilled vegetables for a complete meal.

9. Stir-Fry:

Stir-fry dishes, common in Asian cuisine, are a quick and healthy option for lunch or dinner. A combination of thinly sliced vegetables and your choice of protein is stir-fried in a flavorful sauce, making it a great option for those looking for a balanced meal.

10. Vegetarian and Vegan Options:

As dietary preferences evolve, there's an increasing focus on vegetarian and vegan options for lunch and dinner. Dishes like plant-based burgers, vegan lasagna, and tofu stir-fry offer delicious alternatives for those who choose to avoid meat and animal products.

These lunch and dinner favorites represent just a fraction of the culinary diversity that can be explored. Whether you're looking for quick, satisfying options or are in the mood for a gourmet experience, there's a world of flavors waiting to be discovered in these two essential meals.

Grilled Lemon Herb Chicken

Grilled Lemon Herb Chicken is a delectable and healthy choice for lunch or dinner. This dish combines the natural flavors of succulent chicken with the bright and refreshing zest of lemon, as well as the aromatic and savory notes of various herbs. The result is a meal that is not only delicious but also a perfect representation of balanced and wholesome cooking.

Ingredients for Grilled Lemon Herb Chicken:

1. Chicken: Choose boneless, skinless chicken breasts or thighs for this dish. They are lean and absorb the flavors well.

2. Lemon: Freshly squeezed lemon juice and lemon zest provide a tangy and zesty kick to the dish. The acidity of the lemon helps tenderize the chicken while imparting a bright and citrusy flavor.

3. Herbs: A blend of fresh herbs such as rosemary, thyme, oregano, and parsley adds layers of earthy and aromatic notes to the chicken.

4. Olive Oil: Extra virgin olive oil serves as a base for the marinade, contributing to the chicken's tenderness and providing a rich, smooth texture to the meat.

5. Garlic: Minced garlic cloves infuse the chicken with a deep, savory flavor, complementing the bright lemon and herb components.

6. Salt and Pepper: These two simple seasonings enhance the overall taste of the dish, allowing the other ingredients to shine.

Preparation and Cooking:

1. Marinating the Chicken: Start by preparing the marinade. In a mixing bowl, combine the lemon juice, lemon zest, olive oil, minced garlic, finely chopped herbs, salt, and pepper. Mix these ingredients together to create a flavorful marinade.

2. Coating the Chicken: Place the chicken pieces in a resealable plastic bag or a shallow dish. Pour the marinade over the chicken, ensuring that each piece is well-coated. Seal the bag or cover the dish and refrigerate for at least 30 minutes. Marinating the chicken for a longer period, such as a few hours, allows the flavors to penetrate even further.

3. Grilling: Preheat your grill to medium-high heat. Remove the chicken from the marinade and let any excess liquid drip off. Place the chicken on the grill, cooking for approximately 6-8 minutes on each side, or until the internal temperature reaches 165°F (74°C). The chicken should have beautiful grill marks and a slightly charred appearance.

4. Resting: After grilling, let the chicken rest for a few minutes. This allows the juices to redistribute within the meat, ensuring a moist and tender result.

5. Serving: Slice the grilled lemon herb chicken into portions and garnish with extra lemon wedges and fresh herbs for a burst of color and flavor. This dish pairs well with a variety of sides, such as roasted vegetables, couscous, or a fresh green salad.

Grilled Lemon Herb Chicken is a perfect combination of fresh and vibrant flavors. The citrusy tang of lemon, the earthy aroma of herbs, and the tender juiciness of the grilled chicken make it a favorite for those seeking a healthy and satisfying meal. Whether enjoyed as a summer barbecue delight or a cozy winter dinner, this dish never fails to impress with its simple yet elegant appeal.

Juicy Ribeye Steak with Garlic Butter

Juicy Ribeye Steak with Garlic Butter is a mouthwatering and indulgent favorite for both lunch and dinner. This dish celebrates the rich, beefy flavor of a well-marbled ribeye steak, perfectly cooked to your preferred level of doneness, and then elevated to a whole new level of deliciousness with a decadent garlic butter sauce. It's a classic choice for steak enthusiasts and those looking to treat themselves to a truly satisfying meal.

Ingredients for Juicy Ribeye Steak with Garlic Butter:

1. Ribeye Steak: The star of the show, the ribeye steak, is known for its excellent marbling, which adds a luxurious richness and juiciness to the meat. Choose a thick-cut ribeye for the best results.

2. Salt and Pepper: Simple seasonings of kosher salt and freshly ground black pepper enhance the natural flavors of the steak.

3. Garlic Butter: The garlic butter sauce is made by melting unsalted butter and infusing it with minced garlic. It adds a creamy, savory, and aromatic element to the dish.

4. Fresh Herbs: Optional but delightful additions include fresh herbs like rosemary, thyme, or parsley to garnish the steak and complement the garlic butter.

Preparation and Cooking:

1. Seasoning the Steak: Begin by seasoning the ribeye steak generously with kosher salt and freshly ground black pepper on both sides. Let the steak sit at room temperature for about 30 minutes before cooking to ensure even cooking.

2. Grilling or Pan-Searing: There are two main methods for cooking the ribeye: grilling or pan-searing. If grilling, preheat your grill to high heat. If pan-searing, use a heavy skillet or cast-iron pan over high heat. Either way, you want a hot cooking surface.

3. Cooking the Steak: Place the seasoned ribeye on the grill or in the hot skillet. For medium-rare, cook for about 3-4 minutes on each side, adjusting the time based on your desired level of doneness (medium, medium-well, or well-done).

4. Resting: After cooking, remove the steak from the grill or skillet and let it rest for a few minutes on a cutting board. This step is crucial as it allows the juices to redistribute, ensuring a tender and juicy result.

5. Making the Garlic Butter: While the steak is resting, melt unsalted butter in a small saucepan over low heat. Add minced garlic and let it cook for a minute or two until fragrant. Remove from heat, and your garlic butter is ready.

6. Serving: Slice the ribeye steak into thick, succulent portions and drizzle the garlic butter over the top. Garnish with fresh herbs for a burst of color and an extra layer of flavor. This dish pairs perfectly with sides like mashed potatoes, grilled asparagus, or a simple garden salad.

Juicy Ribeye Steak with Garlic Butter is the epitome of a luxurious and satisfying meal. The tender, well-seasoned ribeye, perfectly seared and accompanied by the rich and aromatic garlic butter, creates a harmonious balance of flavors and textures. It's a classic choice for a special occasion or when you're in the mood for a hearty and indulgent lunch or dinner that's sure to impress.

Creamy Caesar Salad with Grilled Shrimp

Creamy Caesar Salad with Grilled Shrimp is a delightful and elegant choice for lunch or dinner. This dish combines the crisp freshness of a classic Caesar salad with the succulent and smoky flavors of grilled shrimp. The result is a harmonious blend of textures and tastes, making it a favorite for those who crave a combination of creamy, crunchy, and savory elements in their meal.

Ingredients for Creamy Caesar Salad with Grilled Shrimp:

For the Salad:

1. Romaine Lettuce: Fresh, crisp Romaine lettuce forms the base of the salad, providing a satisfying crunch and a mild, slightly bitter flavor.

2. Croutons: Croutons add a delightful, toasty crunch to the salad. You can use store-bought croutons or make your own by toasting bread cubes with olive oil and seasonings.

3. Parmesan Cheese: Grated Parmesan cheese brings a nutty, salty richness to the salad, which complements the creamy Caesar dressing.

For the Caesar Dressing:

4. Mayonnaise: Mayonnaise forms the creamy base of the dressing and contributes to its rich, velvety texture.

5. Anchovy Paste: A small amount of anchovy paste provides a unique umami depth to the dressing, without an overpowering fishy taste.

6. Dijon Mustard: Dijon mustard adds a tangy kick and emulsifies the dressing, creating a smooth consistency.

7. Lemon Juice: Freshly squeezed lemon juice provides a bright and zesty element to balance the creaminess.

8. Garlic: Minced garlic cloves infuse the dressing with a robust and savory flavor.

9. Olive Oil: Extra virgin olive oil enhances the creaminess and smoothness of the dressing.

10. Salt and Pepper: Simple seasonings of salt and freshly ground black pepper allow the other ingredients to shine.

For the Grilled Shrimp:

11. Shrimp: Choose large, peeled, and deveined shrimp for easy preparation. They should be marinated in a simple mixture of olive oil, minced garlic, lemon juice, salt, and pepper before grilling.

Preparation and Assembly:

1. Prepare the Caesar Dressing: In a bowl, whisk together mayonnaise, anchovy paste, Dijon mustard, lemon juice, minced garlic, and olive oil. Season with salt and pepper to taste. Set aside.

2. Grill the Shrimp: Preheat your grill to medium-high heat. Thread the marinated shrimp onto skewers and grill for 2-3 minutes on each side or until they turn pink and opaque.

3. Assemble the Salad: In a large salad bowl, toss the Romaine lettuce with the Caesar dressing until well coated. Add croutons and grated Parmesan cheese and toss again.

4. Add Grilled Shrimp: Carefully place the grilled shrimp on top of the Caesar salad.

5. Serve: Garnish with additional grated Parmesan cheese and a squeeze of fresh lemon juice for an extra burst of flavor. This dish can be served immediately.

Creamy Caesar Salad with Grilled Shrimp is a delightful combination of flavors and textures. The creamy, tangy dressing pairs beautifully with the fresh crunch of the Romaine lettuce, while the grilled shrimp adds a smoky, savory element that takes this classic salad to a whole new level. It's a perfect choice for a light and satisfying lunch or a more substantial dinner, especially when you're in the mood for a restaurant-quality dish at home.

Chapter 5: Sides, Sauces, and Snacks

Sides, sauces, and snacks are the unsung heroes of the culinary world. While the spotlight often shines on main courses, these elements play a crucial role in enhancing the overall dining experience. They add depth, flavor, and texture to a meal, transforming it from ordinary to extraordinary. Whether you're a professional chef or a home cook, understanding the art of sides, sauces, and snacks can take your culinary skills to new heights.

Sides: The Perfect Complement

Sides, also known as side dishes, are essential components of a well-rounded meal. They serve multiple purposes, such as providing balance to a plate, adding nutritional value, and enhancing the overall flavor profile. Some classic side dishes include mashed potatoes, steamed vegetables, and coleslaw, but the possibilities are endless.

The key to great sides lies in their ability to harmonize with the main course. They should complement and contrast with the flavors, textures, and colors of the primary dish. For example, a rich, creamy mashed potato side can balance a spicy Cajun chicken, while a crisp and tangy coleslaw can provide a refreshing contrast to a smoky barbecue brisket.

To elevate your side game, experiment with various cooking techniques and ingredients. Roasting vegetables with olive oil and herbs can create a caramelized, earthy flavor. Grains like quinoa, farro, or couscous can be transformed into hearty and nutritious side dishes with the right seasoning and preparation.

Sauces: The Flavor Enhancers

Sauces are the secret weapons of many chefs, capable of turning a simple dish into a culinary masterpiece. They can be used to add moisture, enhance flavors, or even rescue a seemingly overcooked main course. Whether it's a classic béarnaise sauce for steak or a zesty tomato sauce for pasta, sauces are the bridge that connects all the elements on a plate.

Sauce-making is both an art and a science. It involves the careful balance of flavors, textures, and consistency. From the mother sauces of French cuisine (such as béchamel and velouté) to the complex reductions and emulsions found in haute cuisine, the world of sauces is vast and versatile.

Home cooks can explore the world of sauces by starting with the basics. Simple pan sauces made from the drippings of a roasted chicken or seared steak are accessible options. Classic pasta sauces like marinara or Alfredo can be prepared at home with fresh ingredients. And if you're feeling adventurous, delve into the realms of Asian cuisine with soy-based teriyaki or Thai peanut sauces.

Snacks: The Versatile Delights

Snacks, often considered casual indulgences, have evolved far beyond the realm of chips and pretzels. Today, snacks can be elevated to gourmet status, offering an array of flavors and textures that rival full meals. They serve as the perfect accompaniment to a movie night, a gathering of friends, or a quick pick-me-up during a busy day.

Snacking has taken on a more sophisticated and health-conscious dimension in recent years. Instead of processed junk food, many people now opt for healthier options like roasted nuts, fresh fruit, or artisanal cheeses. Snack boards or platters, adorned with a colorful assortment of goodies, have become a popular way to explore different tastes and textures.

Creating exceptional snacks is all about balance and variety. A well-constructed cheese board, for example, might feature a combination of hard and soft cheeses, fresh and dried fruits, nuts, olives, and a selection of bread or crackers. Meanwhile, spiced and flavored popcorn, vegetable chips, and homemade dips can provide a delightful mix of crunch and flavor.

Sides, sauces, and snacks are essential components of a well-rounded culinary experience. They can turn an ordinary meal into a memorable one, offering a symphony of flavors, textures, and creativity. As a cook, whether amateur or professional, mastering the art of sides, sauces, and snacks can help you elevate your culinary expertise and leave a lasting impression on your guests or customers. So, don't underestimate the power of these culinary elements – they are the true enhancers of every dining experience.

Creamed Spinach with Parmesan

Creamed spinach with Parmesan is a classic side dish that exemplifies the perfect marriage of flavors and textures. This creamy, cheesy creation is a delightful accompaniment to a variety of main courses, from juicy steaks to roasted chicken. The rich, velvety texture of the creamed spinach pairs beautifully with the sharp and nutty notes of Parmesan cheese, making it a favorite among both home cooks and fine dining establishments.

Ingredients for Creamed Spinach with Parmesan:

1. 1 pound fresh spinach leaves, washed and trimmed.
2. 2 tablespoons butter.
3. 2 cloves garlic, minced.
4. 1/4 cup finely chopped onion.
5. 1 cup heavy cream.
6. 1/2 cup grated Parmesan cheese.
7. Salt and freshly ground black pepper to taste.
8. A pinch of freshly grated nutmeg (optional).

Instructions:

1. Prepare the Spinach:

Begin by washing and trimming the fresh spinach leaves. If you prefer a milder flavor, you can remove the tough stems.

2. Sauté the Aromatics:

In a large skillet, melt the butter over medium heat. Add the minced garlic and finely chopped onion. Sauté them until they become translucent and fragrant, about 2-3 minutes.

3. Add the Spinach:

Gradually add the fresh spinach leaves to the skillet. You may need to do this in batches, as the spinach wilts quickly. Stir and cook until the spinach is completely wilted and any excess liquid has evaporated, approximately 3-5 minutes.

4. Prepare the Cream Mixture:

In a separate saucepan, heat the heavy cream over low heat until it begins to warm but not boil. Add the grated Parmesan cheese and stir until it melts into the cream, creating a smooth and creamy sauce. Season the mixture with salt, freshly ground black pepper, and a pinch of freshly grated nutmeg if desired. The nutmeg adds a subtle, warm depth to the dish.

5. Combine the Spinach and Cream:

Pour the Parmesan cream sauce over the sautéed spinach in the skillet. Stir everything together until the spinach is well coated with the creamy mixture.

6. Simmer and Serve:

Let the creamed spinach simmer for a few minutes to allow the flavors to meld and the sauce to thicken slightly. Taste and adjust the seasoning if needed.

7. Garnish and Serve:

Before serving, you can sprinkle a little extra Parmesan cheese on top for an added layer of flavor and a pleasing presentation. Creamed spinach with Parmesan is best served hot, and it makes a fantastic side dish for a variety of main courses.

This dish beautifully balances the earthy, tender spinach with the richness of the cream and the savory, salty notes of Parmesan cheese. The result is a side dish that's both comforting and sophisticated, making it an excellent addition to your culinary repertoire. Creamed spinach with Parmesan is a versatile accompaniment that will undoubtedly elevate your dining experience. Whether served at a formal dinner or a family meal, it's sure to be a crowd-pleaser.

Homemade Beef Jerky

Beef jerky is a timeless snack that has been enjoyed for centuries. This portable, protein-packed treat is perfect for on-the-go adventures, a quick energy boost, or simply as a flavorful and satisfying snack at any time. Making homemade beef jerky allows you to control the quality of the ingredients and experiment with your own unique flavors, ensuring a delicious and personalized snacking experience.

Ingredients for Homemade Beef Jerky:

1. 1 pound of lean beef (such as flank steak or sirloin).

2. 1/4 cup soy sauce or tamari for a gluten-free option.

3. 2 tablespoons Worcestershire sauce.

4. 2 tablespoons of honey or brown sugar.

5. 1 teaspoon garlic powder.

6. 1 teaspoon onion powder.

7. 1/2 teaspoon black pepper.

8. 1/2 teaspoon smoked paprika (for added depth of flavor, optional).

9. 1/4 teaspoon cayenne pepper (adjust to taste for spiciness).

Instructions:

1. Select and Prepare the Meat:

Choose a lean cut of beef and slice it into thin strips, approximately 1/8 to 1/4 inch thick. For the best results, it's easier to slice the meat when it's partially frozen.

2. Marinate the Beef:

In a bowl, combine the soy sauce or tamari, Worcestershire sauce, honey or brown sugar, garlic powder, onion powder, black pepper, smoked paprika, and cayenne pepper. Mix the ingredients to create a flavorful marinade. Place the sliced beef into a resealable plastic bag or a shallow dish, and pour the marinade over it. Seal the bag or cover the dish and refrigerate for at least 2 hours, or overnight for the best results. This step infuses the beef with the delicious flavors.

3. Preheat the Oven or Dehydrator:

Preheat your oven to the lowest temperature setting, typically around 170°F (77°C). If you have a food dehydrator, follow the manufacturer's instructions for beef jerky.

4. Prepare the Meat for Drying:

Remove the marinated beef from the refrigerator and blot it with paper towels to remove excess marinade. The meat should be damp but not dripping wet. This helps speed up the drying process.

5. Dry the Beef:

Arrange the meat strips on oven racks or dehydrator trays. Make sure they are spaced apart to allow for proper air circulation. For oven drying, prop the oven door open slightly with a wooden spoon to help moisture escape. Allow the beef to dry for 4-6 hours, or until it reaches your desired level of dryness and chewiness. You can periodically check the jerky's progress during the drying process.

6. Cool and Store:

Once the beef jerky is done, let it cool completely. It should be firm and not overly pliable. Store it in an airtight container or vacuum-sealed bag to maintain freshness.

Homemade beef jerky offers a world of customization. You can experiment with different marinades and spices to create your signature flavors, whether you prefer sweet, spicy, smoky, or tangy. The result is a high-protein, low-fat snack that's perfect for hiking, road trips, or simply enjoying at home.

By making your own beef jerky, you can control the quality of the meat and ingredients, ensuring a healthier and tastier snack option compared to many store-bought versions. It's a rewarding culinary endeavor that can be as simple or complex as you like, providing you with a snack that's not only delicious but also made with your personal touch.

Carnivore-Friendly Dipping Sauces

While carnivores predominantly focus on animal products for their diet, that doesn't mean their meals have to be devoid of flavor and variety. Carnivore-friendly dipping sauces provide a delightful way to enhance the flavors of meat-based dishes, adding a burst of excitement to every bite. These sauces can be enjoyed with a wide range of meats, from grilled steaks to roasted poultry and everything in between.

Here are some delicious and meat-centric dipping sauces that can elevate your carnivore dining experience:

1. Garlic Butter Sauce:

Garlic butter sauce is a timeless classic that pairs wonderfully with grilled or pan-seared meats. To make this savory delight, you'll need:

- 1/2 cup of unsalted butter.
- 4-5 cloves of garlic, minced.
- Salt and black pepper to taste.
- A squeeze of fresh lemon juice (optional).

Instructions:

  - Melt the butter in a saucepan over low heat.
  - Add the minced garlic and sauté for a minute or two until fragrant.
  - Season with salt, black pepper, and a squeeze of fresh lemon juice for a zesty twist.
  - Serve the garlic butter sauce hot, drizzled over your favorite meat.

2. Chimichurri Sauce:

Chimichurri is a zesty and herbaceous sauce that originated in Argentina. It's a fantastic accompaniment for grilled beef, lamb, or chicken. For a carnivore-friendly version, use high-quality beef fat in place of oil. Here's what you'll need:

- 1 cup of fresh parsley, finely chopped.
- 1/4 cup of fresh oregano, finely chopped.
- 2-3 cloves of garlic, minced.
- 1/2 cup of rendered beef fat (lard).
- Red pepper flakes to taste.
- Salt and black pepper to taste.
- 2 tablespoons of red wine vinegar (optional).

Instructions:

- Mix the chopped parsley, oregano, and minced garlic in a bowl.
- Add the rendered beef fat, red pepper flakes, salt, and black pepper.
- If desired, include a splash of red wine vinegar for acidity.
- Allow the flavors to meld for a few minutes before serving with your grilled meats.

3. Blue Cheese Dipping Sauce:

Blue cheese lovers will relish this creamy and tangy dipping sauce, perfect for pairing with a succulent steak or roasted meats. Gather these ingredients:

- 1/2 cup of heavy cream.
- 1/2 cup of crumbled blue cheese.
- 1 tablespoon of butter.
- Salt and black pepper to taste.

Instructions:

- In a small saucepan, warm the heavy cream over low heat.
- Stir in the crumbled blue cheese and butter, allowing them to melt and create a creamy consistency.
- Season with salt and black pepper to taste.
- Serve the blue cheese sauce hot, and drizzle it over your cooked meat.

These carnivore-friendly dipping sauces not only enhance the taste of your meat-based dishes but also provide a welcome change of pace. Whether you prefer the rich, buttery notes of garlic butter, the bold flavors of chimichurri, or the creamy tang of blue cheese, these sauces are versatile, easy to prepare, and sure to satisfy carnivores and flavor enthusiasts alike. So, fire up the grill or sear your favorite cuts, and get ready to take your carnivore meals to the next level with these delectable dipping sauces.

Chapter 6: Sweet and Savory Treats

Sweet and savory treats are a delightful category of culinary creations that tantalize the taste buds with their combination of contrasting flavors. These treats offer a unique blend of sweetness and saltiness, creating a harmonious balance that appeals to a wide range of palates. Whether you're a fan of traditional desserts or prefer something more unconventional, sweet and savory treats offer endless possibilities for culinary experimentation.

One of the most iconic examples of a sweet and savory treat is the classic combination of salted caramel. The rich, buttery sweetness of caramel is enhanced by a pinch of salt, creating a flavor profile that's both comforting and exciting. Salted caramel can be used in a variety of desserts, from ice cream and brownies to drizzled on top of popcorn. Its popularity has made it a staple in modern dessert menus around the world.

Another beloved sweet and savory pairing is the fusion of cheese and fruit. The creaminess of cheese, whether it's a mild brie or a sharp cheddar, complements the natural sweetness of fruits like figs, apples, and pears. Cheese platters often feature a combination of these elements, creating a delightful contrast in flavors and textures. Whether enjoyed as an appetizer or a dessert, cheese and fruit pairings are sure to please the palate.

For those who enjoy a bit of heat with their sweets, chili-infused chocolate is a bold choice. The spicy kick of chili peppers can be incorporated into chocolate bars, truffles, or even hot chocolate, creating a unique and memorable flavor experience. The combination of sweet and spicy in these treats adds an exciting dimension to your taste sensations.

Savory treats with a sweet twist also have a special place in the culinary world. One such example is maple-glazed bacon. The smoky, savory flavor of bacon is elevated to new heights when it's coated with a sweet, sticky maple syrup glaze. The result is a mouthwatering combination of crispy, salty, and sweet that's perfect for breakfast or as a snack.

Pretzels are another versatile component in the world of sweet and savory treats. They can be transformed from a traditional salty snack into a sweet delight by dipping them in chocolate or caramel. The contrast between the crunchy, salty pretzel and the smooth, sweet coating is an irresistible combination.

The fusion of sweet and savory flavors can be found in various global cuisines as well. In Asian cuisine, dishes like teriyaki chicken or Thai pineapple fried rice often feature a balance of sweet and savory flavors, incorporating ingredients like soy sauce, sugar, and fresh fruits. These dishes demonstrate how sweet and savory can coexist harmoniously in a single meal.

The versatility of sweet and savory treats extends to both simple home creations and elaborate restaurant offerings. They provide an exciting playground for culinary experimentation and innovation. Whether you're craving a delightful dessert or a unique appetizer, exploring the world of sweet and savory treats can lead to unexpected flavor combinations that are sure to satisfy your taste buds and leave you craving more.

Beef and Bacon Fat Bombs

Sweet and savory treats come in many delectable forms, and one of the most indulgent and satisfying options is the "Beef and Bacon Fat Bomb." This unique creation combines the richness of beef and bacon with a sweet twist, resulting in a mouthwatering combination that's sure to please those who enjoy a hearty and unconventional treat.

Ingredients for Beef and Bacon Fat Bombs:

1. Ground Beef: Use lean ground beef for a healthier option, or opt for fattier cuts for a more indulgent experience.

2. Bacon: Choose crispy bacon, as it adds a savory, smoky flavor to the fat bombs.

3. Cream Cheese: Cream cheese serves as the creamy, tangy component that balances the flavors.

4. Sweetener: A low-carb sweetener, such as erythritol or stevia, is used to add a touch of sweetness to the fat bombs.

5. Spices: Seasonings like garlic powder, onion powder, and black pepper enhance the savory elements of the dish.

6. Chopped Herbs: Fresh herbs like parsley, chives, or rosemary can be used for added freshness and aroma.

Instructions:

1. Cook the Bacon: Begin by cooking the bacon until it's crispy and golden. Once done, remove it from the pan and allow it to cool. Afterward, crumble or chop it into small bits.

2. Sauté the Ground Beef: In the same pan with the bacon grease, cook the ground beef until it's browned and cooked through. Drain any excess fat if necessary, but retain some for flavor.

3. Combine Beef and Bacon: In a mixing bowl, combine the cooked ground beef and crumbled bacon. Mix them thoroughly to ensure an even distribution of flavors.

4. Prepare the Sweet and Savory Mixture: Add the cream cheese to the beef and bacon mixture, along with the sweetener and spices. Mix everything well until you have a creamy, savory filling.

5. Shape the Fat Bombs: Using a spoon or your hands, shape the mixture into small, bite-sized fat bombs. You can form them into balls or any shape you prefer.

6. Chill: Place the fat bombs on a baking sheet and refrigerate them for at least an hour or until they firm up. This chilling process will make them easier to handle and serve.

7. Garnish: Before serving, you can garnish your beef and bacon fat bombs with freshly chopped herbs to add a burst of fresh aroma and a pop of color.

These beef and bacon fat bombs are a delightful blend of savory and sweet. The bacon and beef provide a rich, umami depth of flavor, while the cream cheese and sweetener add a subtle sweetness that balances the overall taste. The result is a satisfying and indulgent treat that can be enjoyed as a snack or even as a unique appetizer at your next gathering.

It's important to note that these fat bombs are low in carbohydrates and high in fat, making them a popular choice for those following a ketogenic or low-carb diet. They offer a delicious way to incorporate healthy fats into your diet while satisfying your cravings for both sweet and savory flavors. So, the next time you're looking for a unique treat that pushes the boundaries of flavor, give beef and bacon fat bombs a try, and experience the best of both worlds in a single bite.

Chocolate-Covered Bacon

Chocolate-covered bacon is a delightful and unconventional sweet and savory treat that combines the smoky, salty goodness of bacon with the smooth and decadent sweetness of chocolate. This culinary creation has gained popularity in recent years, and for good reason – it's a tantalizing blend of flavors and textures that appeals to those with a penchant for unique and adventurous snacks.

Ingredients for Chocolate-Covered Bacon:

1. Bacon Strips: You can use either crispy cooked bacon or partially cooked bacon, depending on your preference.

2. Chocolate: High-quality chocolate, whether dark, milk, or white, is the key to achieving a delectable result. Choose your favorite chocolate for the perfect coating.

3. Optional Toppings: You can further enhance your chocolate-covered bacon by adding toppings like crushed nuts, sea salt, or even a dusting of powdered sugar.

Instructions:

1. Cook the Bacon: Begin by cooking the bacon until it's crispy and golden brown. You can use your preferred method, such as frying in a pan or baking in the oven. Let the bacon cool on a paper towel to remove excess grease.

2. Prepare the Chocolate: In a microwave-safe bowl or on the stovetop using a double boiler, melt the chocolate slowly and gently, stirring to ensure it's smooth and glossy.

3. Dip the Bacon: Take each strip of bacon and dip it into the melted chocolate, ensuring that it's well-coated. You can choose to coat the entire strip or just half, depending on your preference.

4. Place on a Baking Sheet: After dipping, place the chocolate-covered bacon on a baking sheet lined with parchment paper. This will prevent the bacon from sticking and make cleanup easier.

5. Add Toppings (Optional): While the chocolate is still soft, you can sprinkle your chosen toppings onto the chocolate-covered bacon. Popular choices include crushed nuts, a touch of sea salt, or a dusting of powdered sugar.

6. Chill: Once all the bacon strips are coated and garnished, place the baking sheet in the refrigerator to allow the chocolate to harden. This will take around 30 minutes to an hour.

7. Serve and Enjoy: Once the chocolate has set, your chocolate-covered bacon is ready to be enjoyed. The contrast between the salty, savory bacon and the sweet, luscious chocolate is a delightful taste experience.

Chocolate-covered bacon is a versatile treat that can be customized to suit your preferences. For a classic take, use dark chocolate to create a rich and robust flavor. If you prefer a sweeter contrast, opt for milk chocolate. White chocolate offers a creamier, more delicate sweetness.

The addition of toppings can also elevate the experience. The crunch of nuts, the burst of sea salt, or the subtle sweetness of powdered sugar can all add layers of complexity to the treat.

Whether you serve chocolate-covered bacon as a fun party snack, a unique dessert, or simply as a self-indulgent treat, it's a must-try for those who enjoy the intriguing interplay of sweet and savory flavors. This inventive combination might surprise and delight your taste buds, making it a memorable addition to your culinary repertoire.

Vanilla Almond Panna Cotta

Vanilla almond panna cotta is a luscious and elegant sweet treat that beautifully marries the delicate flavors of vanilla and almonds. This Italian dessert is known for its creamy, silky texture and subtle sweetness, making it a favorite among those who appreciate the harmonious combination of sweet and savory elements. If you're looking for a dessert that's both sophisticated and easy to prepare, vanilla almond panna cotta is an excellent choice.

Ingredients for Vanilla Almond Panna Cotta:

1. Heavy Cream: This is the primary ingredient that gives panna cotta its creamy, indulgent texture.

2. Whole Milk: Whole milk adds richness and creaminess while keeping the dessert from becoming overly heavy.

3. Sugar: Granulated sugar sweetens the dessert, giving it a balanced, delicate sweetness.

4. Vanilla Bean or Extract: The star of the show, vanilla, infuses the panna cotta with its fragrant and comforting flavor.

5. Almond Extract: Almond extract imparts a subtle nutty flavor, enhancing the overall experience.

6. Gelatin: Gelatin is what sets the panna cotta and gives it its signature wobbly texture.

7. Sliced Almonds (optional): Sliced almonds can be added as a garnish for a crunchy texture and added almond flavor.

Instructions:

1. Bloom the Gelatin: Start by placing the gelatin in a small bowl of cold water. Allow it to soak for about 5-10 minutes, or until it becomes soft and pliable.

2. Heat the Cream and Milk: In a saucepan, combine the heavy cream, whole milk, and sugar.

Gently heat the mixture over medium-low heat until it's hot but not boiling. Stir occasionally to dissolve the sugar.

3. Add the Vanilla and Almond Flavors: Split the vanilla bean (if using) and scrape out the seeds. Add the seeds to the cream mixture, or if using vanilla extract, add it at this stage. Also, add the almond extract for a hint of nutty flavor. Remove the saucepan from the heat.

4. Incorporate the Gelatin: Squeeze the excess water from the bloomed gelatin and add it to the cream mixture. Stir until the gelatin is completely dissolved.

5. Strain the Mixture: To ensure a smooth and creamy panna cotta, strain the mixture through a fine-mesh sieve to remove any lumps or vanilla bean pieces.

6. Divide and Chill: Pour the strained mixture into individual serving glasses or ramekins. Allow them to cool at room temperature for a while, then refrigerate for at least 4 hours, or until the panna cotta is set and has a delicate wobble.

7. Serve with Almonds (Optional): Before serving, you can garnish the panna cotta with sliced almonds for an extra layer of flavor and texture.

Vanilla almond panna cotta is a versatile dessert that can be enjoyed on its own or paired with a variety of toppings and accompaniments. Fresh berries, fruit coulis, or a drizzle of honey are all excellent choices to complement the creamy sweetness of the panna cotta.

The balance of the warm, comforting vanilla and the subtle nuttiness of almond extract creates a delightful blend of sweet and savory notes that make this dessert truly memorable. Whether you're hosting a special occasion or simply indulging in a moment of self-pampering, vanilla almond panna cotta is sure to elevate the dining experience and leave a lasting impression on your taste buds.

Seniors' Carnivore Smoothie Bowl

The "Seniors' Carnivore Smoothie Bowl" is a unique and nutritionally rich dish designed with seniors' dietary needs in mind. This innovative take on a classic smoothie bowl is tailored to meet the nutritional requirements of older adults while offering a delightful combination of sweet and savory flavors. As we age, maintaining a well-balanced diet becomes increasingly important, and this bowl provides a satisfying and delicious way to do just that.

Ingredients for Seniors' Carnivore Smoothie Bowl:

1. Lean Protein: Seniors need ample protein to maintain muscle mass and overall health. Lean sources like grilled chicken or turkey breast are great choices.

2. Low-Fat Greek Yogurt: Greek yogurt offers probiotics for gut health and added protein.

3. Fresh Berries: Berries are rich in antioxidants, vitamins, and fiber.

4. Spinach or Kale: Leafy greens like spinach or kale provide essential vitamins and minerals while being easy to digest.

5. Walnuts or Almonds: Nuts are packed with healthy fats and provide a satisfying crunch.

6. Honey or Maple Syrup: These natural sweeteners can add a touch of sweetness to balance the savory elements.

7. Chia or Flax Seeds: These seeds are a great source of fiber and healthy fats, which are beneficial for seniors.

8. Cottage Cheese (Optional): Cottage cheese is high in protein and can enhance the creaminess of the bowl.

Instructions:

1. **Prepare the Protein:** Start by grilling or poaching the chicken or turkey breast until it's fully cooked. Allow it to cool and then slice or dice it into bite-sized pieces.

2. **Create the Smoothie Base:** In a blender, combine low-fat Greek yogurt with a handful of fresh berries, spinach or kale, and a drizzle of honey or maple syrup for sweetness. Blend until you have a smooth and vibrant green base.

3. **Assemble the Bowl:** Pour the smoothie base into a bowl. Top it with the diced chicken or turkey, and then add a generous spoonful of low-fat cottage cheese if you're including it.

4. **Add Crunch:** Sprinkle crushed walnuts or almonds on top of the smoothie bowl. These provide a delightful crunch and healthy fats.

5. **Garnish with Seeds:** Finish the bowl by adding chia or flax seeds. These seeds are not only

visually appealing but also provide extra fiber and nutrition.

6. Serve: The Seniors' Carnivore Smoothie Bowl is ready to be served. It's best enjoyed fresh and can be customized with additional toppings or seasonings to suit individual preferences.

This unique smoothie bowl offers a wealth of nutritional benefits for seniors. The lean protein helps maintain muscle strength, while the low-fat dairy products and nuts contribute to healthy fats and added protein. The inclusion of fresh berries and leafy greens provides essential vitamins, antioxidants, and fiber that are crucial for overall well-being. The natural sweeteners and creamy yogurt make the dish more enjoyable while keeping added sugars in check.

For older adults, maintaining a balanced diet that caters to their specific nutritional needs is vital. The Seniors' Carnivore Smoothie Bowl is a creative way to achieve this balance while offering a delicious blend of sweet and savory flavors. It's a versatile dish that can be adapted to individual dietary requirements and preferences, making it a valuable addition to the senior diet and a delightful treat that promotes both health and enjoyment.

Conclusion

The carnivore diet is a dietary approach that has gained attention for its emphasis on animal-based foods while excluding most plant-based items. Advocates of the carnivore diet claim various health benefits, including weight loss, improved mental clarity, and relief from certain health conditions. However, it's essential to approach this diet with caution and consider both its potential advantages and drawbacks.

While some people may experience short-term benefits from the carnivore diet, such as weight loss and symptom relief, the long-term health implications are less clear. The diet's extreme restriction of plant foods can lead to deficiencies in essential vitamins, minerals, and dietary fiber, which are crucial for overall health. Additionally, the diet's impact on cholesterol levels and heart health remains a topic of debate among experts.

It is important to consult with a healthcare professional or registered dietitian before embarking on the carnivore diet or any extreme dietary plan. Individual nutritional needs vary, and what works for one person may not be suitable for another. A balanced diet that incorporates a wide variety of foods, including fruits, vegetables, lean proteins, and whole grains, is generally recommended for long-term health and well-being.

The carnivore diet is a restrictive and controversial eating plan that should be approached with caution. It may offer some short-term benefits for certain individuals, but the potential long-term risks and nutritional deficiencies need to be carefully considered. A balanced and varied diet, tailored to individual needs, remains a more widely accepted approach for promoting overall health and wellness.